Blood Pressure Breakthrough

Your Path to Hypertension Control

Rossana Lewis

Thank you for purchasing my book. I'd really appreciate if you could take a moment to leave a review on amazon. Your feedback will help me improve and make my next book even better. I'm always looking for ways to improve, so please do not hold back! Thank you for your time and support.

TABLE OF CONTENT

Chapter 1: Understanding High Blood Pressure

1.1 What is High Blood Pressure (Hypertension)?

High blood pressure, also known as hypertension, is when your blood pressure, the force of your blood pushing against the walls of your blood vessels, is consistently too high. To survive and function properly, your tissues and organs need the oxygenated blood that your circulatory system carries throughout the body. When the heart beats, it creates pressure that pushes blood through a network of tube-shaped blood vessels, which include arteries, veins and capillaries. This pressure — blood pressure — is the result of two forces: The first force (systolic pressure) occurs as blood pumps out of the heart and into the arteries that are part of the circulatory system. The second force (diastolic pressure) is created as the heart rests between heart beats. These two forces are each represented by numbers in a blood pressure reading. The primary way that high blood pressure causes harm is by increasing the workload of the heart and blood vessels — making them work harder and less efficiently.

Over time, the force and friction of high blood pressure damages the delicate tissues inside the arteries. In turn, LDL (bad) cholesterol forms plaque along tiny tears in the artery walls, signifying the start of atherosclerosis.

The more the plaque and damage increases, the narrower the insides of the arteries become —

raising blood pressure and starting a vicious circle that further harms your arteries, heart and the rest of your body. This can ultimately lead to other conditions ranging from arrhythmia to heart attack and stroke.

You may not feel that anything is wrong, but high blood pressure could be quietly causing damage that can threaten your health. The best prevention is knowing your numbers and making changes that matter in order to prevent or manage high blood pressure.

1.2 The Silent Threat: Why Hypertension Matters

About 1 in 3 adults in the U.S. has high blood pressure, but many don't realize it. High blood pressure is sometimes called a "silent killer," because it usually has no warning signs, yet it can lead to life-threatening conditions like heart attack or stroke. The good news is that high blood pressure, or hypertension, can often be prevented or treated. Early diagnosis and simple, healthy changes can keep high blood pressure from seriously damaging your health.

Normal blood flow delivers nutrients and oxygen to all parts of your body, including important organs like your heart, brain, and kidneys. Your beating heart helps to push blood through your vast network of blood vessels, both large and small. Your blood vessels, in turn, constantly adjust. They become narrower or wider to maintain your blood pressure and keep blood flowing at a healthy rate.

It's normal for your blood pressure to go up and down throughout each day. Blood pressure is affected by time of day, exercise, the foods you eat, stress, and other factors. Problems can arise, though, if your blood pressure stays too high for too long.

High blood pressure can make your heart work too hard and lose strength. The high force of blood flow can damage your blood vessels, making them weak, stiff, or narrower. Over time, hypertension can harm several important organs, including your heart, kidneys, brain, and eyes.

Anyone, even children, can develop high blood pressure. But the risk for hypertension rises with age. Once people are in their 60s, about two-thirds of the population is affected by hypertension. Excess weight or having a family history of high blood pressure also raises your risk for hypertension.

African Americans are especially likely to get hypertension. Compared to Caucasian or Hispanic American adults, African Americans tend to develop hypertension at a younger age and to have a higher blood pressure on average.

Because it usually has no symptoms, the only way to know for sure that you have hypertension is to have a blood pressure test. This easy, painless test involves placing an inflated cuff with a pressure gauge around your upper arm to squeeze the blood vessels. A health care provider may then use a stethoscope to listen to your pulse as air is released from the cuff, or an automatic device may measure the pressure. Blood pressure is given as 2 numbers. The first number represents the pressure in your blood vessels as the heart beats (called systolic pressure). The second is the pressure as your heart relaxes and fills with blood (diastolic pressure). Experts generally agree that the safest blood pressure—or "normal" blood pressure—is 120/80 or lower, meaning systolic blood pressure is 120 or less and diastolic pressure is 80 or less. If your blood pressure falls between "normal" and "hypertension," it's sometimes called prehypertension. People with prehypertension are more likely to end up with high blood pressure if they don't take steps to prevent it.

If you're diagnosed with high blood pressure, your doctor will prescribe a treatment plan. You'll likely be advised to make healthy lifestyle changes. You may also need to take medications. The goal of treatment is to reduce your blood pressure enough to avoid more serious problems.

How low should you aim when reducing your blood pressure? The answer depends on many factors, which is why it's important to work with your doctor on blood pressure goals. Most current guidelines recommend aiming for a systolic pressure below 140. These medical guidelines are sometimes adjusted as new research is reported.

1.3 Types and Stages of High Blood Pressure

There are different types of hypertension which can affect anyone.

Primary Hypertension (also known as Essential Hypertension): For almost 90% of the patients, the cause of this Hypertension is unknown. Your doctor will diagnose this Hypertension type after analyzing your blood pressure after three or four visits. People who suffer from this Hypertension type show no significant symptoms. However, a few patients do show the below signs:

- Frequent headaches
- Fatigue
- Dizziness
- Nosebleeds

Secondary Hypertension: This Hypertension type occurs when there is an abnormality in the arteries that supply blood to the kidneys.

Some common causes of this Hypertension include:

- Abnormalities or tumours of the adrenal glands
- Thyroid
- Hormonal imbalances
- Excessive salt or alcohol intake

Malignant Hypertension: Here the blood pressure rises rather quickly and causes a medical emergency where the patient needs to be rushed to the hospital. It is typically observed in small fractions of society such as young African-American men and women with pregnancy toxaemia, to name a few.

Some common symptoms include:

- Numbness in arms and legs
- A headache
- Chest pain
- Blurry vision

Resistant Hypertension: This type of Hypertension is usually observed in people who are aged, obese or are suffering from diabetes or kidney ailments.

Now, let's talk about it's stages. Under the new 2017 guidelines, all blood pressure measurements over 120/80 mm Hg are considered elevated. Now blood pressure measurements are categorized as follows:

- Normal: systolic less than 120 mm Hg and diastolic less than 80 mm Hg
- Elevated: systolic between 120-129 mm Hg and diastolic less than 80 mm Hg
- Stage 1: systolic between 130-139 mm Hg or diastolic between 80-89 mm Hg
- Stage 2: systolic at least 140 mm Hg or diastolic at least 90 mm Hg.

The new classification system puts more people into the elevated category who were previously considered prehypertension. Under the new guidelines,an estimated 46 percent of U.S. adults became categorized as having high blood pressure. Treatment is recommended at the elevated stage if you have heart disease or other risk factors, such as diabetes and family health history. If your blood pressure reading is in the elevated category, discuss with your doctor what steps you can take to lower it.

Chapter 2: The Mechanics of Blood Pressure

2.1 How Blood Pressure is Measured

A blood pressure reading is usually taken while a person is seated in a chair with the feet flat on the floor. The arm should rest comfortably at heart level. The blood pressure cuff goes around the top part of the arm. The bottom of the cuff is just above the elbow. It's important that the cuff fits. Blood pressure readings can vary if the cuff is too big or too small.

Blood pressure readings can be taken with the help of a machine. This is called an automated measurement. When a machine isn't used, this is called a manual measurement. For a manual blood pressure measurement, the care provider places a stethoscope over the major artery in the upper arm (brachial artery) to listen to blood flow. The cuff is inflated with a small hand pump. As the cuff inflates, it squeezes the arm. Blood flow through the artery stops for a moment. The health care provider opens a valve on the hand pump to slowly release the air in the cuff and restore blood flow. The provider continues to listen to blood flow and pulse and records the blood pressure.

For an automated measurement, the blood pressure cuff automatically inflates and measures the pulse. In this case, a stethoscope is not needed. It takes about one minute to get a blood pressure measurement.

2.2 Blood Pressure Variation

Blood pressure has a daily pattern. Usually, blood pressure starts to rise a few hours before a person wakes up. It continues to rise during the day, peaking in midday. It typically drops in the late afternoon and evening. Blood pressure is usually lower at night while sleeping. The blood pressure measurement at night is called nocturnal blood pressure. Examples of an irregular blood pressure pattern include:

- High blood pressure during the night
- High blood pressure early in the morning
- Less than 10% drop in blood pressure overnight (nondipping blood pressure)

A rise in blood pressure overnight to early morning has been linked to an increased risk of heart disease. An irregular blood pressure pattern could also mean that you have:

- Poorly controlled high blood pressure

- Obstructive sleep apnea

- Kidney disease

- Diabetes

- Thyroid disease

- A nervous system disorder

Poor diet, lack of exercise and certain lifestyle factors can affect blood pressure pattern, including:

- Night-shift work

- Smoking

- Overweight or obesity

- Stress and anxiety

- Not taking medications for blood pressure or sleep apnea as directed, or ineffective treatment.

Your health care provider can tell you if an irregular daily blood pressure pattern needs treatment. Sometimes, a person's blood pressure rises simply when seeing a care provider. This is called whitecoat hypertension.

A 24-hour blood pressure monitoring test can be done to measure blood pressure at regular time periods over 24 hours. The test is called ambulatory blood pressure monitoring. It provides a detailed look at blood pressure changes over an average day and night.

Chapter 3: Causes and Risk Factors

3.1 Genetics and Family History

A family history of high blood pressure means you have someone in your family (a blood relative such as a mother, father, sister, or brother) who has or had high blood pressure before the age of 60. The more family members you have with high blood pressure before the age of 60, the stronger the family history of high blood pressure. High blood pressure tends to run in families for many reasons. Blood relatives tend to have many of the same genes that can predispose a person to high blood pressure, heart disease, or stroke. Genes are units of heredity that are passed from parents to children. Relatives may also share some of the same habits such as diet, exercise, and smoking that can affect risk.

There are several things. You should get your blood pressure checked at least once a year to make sure it is within normal levels. Reduce other risks for high blood pressure by eating healthy foods, using less salt, exercising, losing weight if needed and stopping smoking. If you are already being treated for high blood pressure, it is important to take the medications regularly that have been prescribed for you. Also, keep your scheduled appointments with your health care provider. Finding the best treatment for each person often takes time and what works for one person may not work for another. What is important is that you keep trying to lower your blood pressure with the help of your health care provider!

3.2 Lifestyle Factors

Your lifestyle choices have an impact on your health and well-being in general. From your diet to how you manage stress play a crucial role in determining the quality of life and your risk for various health conditions.

Nutrition is the first you may consider. When you lack some nutrients in the food you eat, it may go a long way in determining your risk for high blood pressure. Sometimes it's always advisable to eat eat fruits, vegetables and a balanced diet to help reduce the risk. Note that food is essential to fight diseases and keep your healthy even if you have a health condition or not, you just need it to keep living.

Also, when you don't keep your body fit by exercising, you may also be proned to this health conditions. Exercising your body makes your heart beats faster which is sometimes needed to pump blood and make it flow to other regions of the body. Making the heartbeat is natural but when it beats more than expected and too frequent then it becomes a problem.

Stress is also another risk factor. You know how stress could have a toll on your mental health, it could also increase your risk of high blood pressure especially if you're obese and not getting the relaxation your body needs.

Tobacco and alcohol increases your risk of high blood pressure too. Excessive intake can also have adverse health effects. If you're addicted to any of these you should try to reduce your intake to the nearest minimum if you want to battle high blood pressure.

3.3 Health Conditions and Hypertension

High blood pressure is also influenced by a number of other health conditions. Let's talk about the relationship between hypertension and other health conditions.

Cardiovascular Disease: Cardiovascular diseases such as coronary artery disease, diseases such as coronary artery disease, congestive heart failure and atrial fibrillation are all related to high blood pressure. Elevated blood pressure can strain the heart and blood vessels increasing the risk of this condition.

Diabetes: Is a companion of hypertension referred to as a silent killer. When diabetes is uncontrolled, it can damage blood vessels thereby increasing the risk of hypertension. While hypertension can worsen diabetes related conditions.

Kidney Disease: Kidneys play a pivotal role in blood regulation which hypertension can damage the delicate blood vessels in the kidneys leading to kidney disease. Conversely, kidney disease can disrupt the body's ability to regulate blood pressure, causing hypertension. One has to manage these conditions as it is essential to prevent further kidney damage.

Obesity: Excess weight in the body, especially abdominal obesity has a strong link with hypertension. More blood supply is required by the additional fat tissue which increases more workload on the heart and blood vessels. Weight loss is a primary strategy for managing hypertension.

Sleep Apnea: Is characterized by breathing disruptions while sleeping. It has a bidirectional relationship with hypertension. It can also contribute to elevated blood pressure and hypertension can as well worsen the symptoms of sleep apnea.

High Cholesterol: Elevated levels of low-density lipoprotein (LDL) cholesterol (bad cholesterol) are related to atherosclerosis, a condition in which fatty deposits accumulate in the arteries. This alone can raise blood pressure and contribute to hypertension.

Thyroid Disorders: Underactive thyroid also known as hypothyroidism and overactive thyroid also known as hyperthyroidism can impact blood pressure. Hypothyroidism can lead to weight gain and elevated cholesterol levels, while hyperthyroidism can accelerate heart rate and increase the risk of atrial fibrillation.

Mental Health: Stress, depression and anxiety can have a direct influence or impact on blood pressure. Having chronic stress can lead to hypertension and worsen already existing blood pressure. Managing mental health through therapy, relaxation techniques and a series of lifestyle changes is crucial in controlling high blood pressure.

Pregnancy-Related Hypertension: There are conditions like gestational hypertension and preeclampsia which can develop during pregnancy. These conditions need careful monitoring and management to ensure the health of both the baby and the mother.

Chapter 4: Signs and Symptoms of Hypertension

4.1 Recognizing Silent Symptoms

One of the most dangerous things about hypertension or high blood pressure is that you may not know you have it. In fact, nearly one-third of people who have high blood pressure don't know it. That's because high blood pressure doesn't have any symptoms unless it's very severe. The best way to know if your blood pressure is high is through regular checkups. You can also monitor blood pressure at home. This is especially important if you have a close relative who has high blood pressure. If your blood pressure is extremely high, there may be certain symptoms to look out for, including:

- Severe headaches

- Nosebleed

- Fatigue or confusion

- Vision problems

- Chest pain

- A hard time breathing

- Irregular heartbeat

- Blood in the urine

- Pounding in your chest, neck, or ears

- Seizures

People sometimes feel that other symptoms may be related to high blood pressure, but they may not be.

4.2 When to Seek Medical Attention

If you have any of these symptoms, see a doctor right away. You could be having a hypertensive crisis that could lead to a heart attack or stroke. You may also have another serious health condition. Most of the time, high blood pressure doesn't cause headaches or nosebleeds. But this can happen in a hypertensive crisis when blood pressure is above 180/120. If your blood pressure is extremely high and you have these symptoms, rest for 5 minutes and check again. If your blood pressure is still unusually high, it's a medical emergency. Call 911.

It's important to remember that high blood pressure doesn't usually have symptoms. So, everyone should get it checked regularly. The American Heart Association recommends adults with normal blood pressure should get blood pressure checked each year at routine health visits. You may also have it checked at a health resource fair or other events or places in your community.

If you have high blood pressure, your doctor might recommend you monitor it more often at home. At-home monitors may work better than store-based machines. Your doctor will also recommend making lifestyle changes along with medications to lower your blood pressure. Untreated hypertension can lead to serious diseases, including stroke, heart disease, kidney failure, and eye problems.

Chapter 5: Lifestyle Modifications

5.1 The Role of Diet in Blood Pressure Control

The role of diet in controlling high blood pressure is crucial. Making the right dietary choices can help reduce your risk and also decrease your need for medications. Now let's explore the role of these diets which helps in blood pressure control.

Sodium (Salt) Reduction: Excessive salt intake is a major contributor to hypertension. Sodium makes the body retain water thereby increasing blood volume and blood pressure as well.

Limiting salt intake to 2,300 milligrams per day and ideally 1,500 for some individuals can help in blood pressure control. Also, reducing food from restaurants and that which is processed and using herbs and spices for flavor can reduce salt intake.

Potassium Intake: Potassium helps neutralize the effect of sodium, relaxing blood vessels walls and reducing blood pressure. One should take potassium rich foods such as potatoes, oranges, spinach, bananas and beans. Aim for around 4,700 milligrams per day.

Magnesium Consumption: Magnesium supports nerve and normal muscle function and the relaxation of blood vessels. Magnesium rich foods include seeds, nuts, grains and leafy greens. Aim for about 4,000 milligrams a day.

Whole Grains and Fiber: Fiber helps in maintaining a healthy weight which is also essential for blood pressure control and may lower cholesterol levels. Incorporate whole grains such as oats, brown rice and wheat in your diet. Aim for at least 25 grams per day.

Healthy Fats: These are found in avocados, fatty fish and olive oil which are monounsaturated and polyunsaturated fats. It is always advisable to choose these fats over saturated and trans fats found in processed and fried foods.

Limit Alcohol Consumption: Too much alcohol intake can lead to hypertension and other cardiovascular problems too. If you need to take alcohol, moderate your intake.

Maintain a Healthy Weight: Abdominal obesity and excess body weight increases the risk of hypertension. Adopt a balanced diet and engage in physical activity so as to achieve a healthy weight.

Manage Stress: Being stressed is healthy when you're engaged but when you're being stressed often then it becomes a problem and can be chronic which raises blood pressure. Stress management techniques are important. To reduce stress, engage in yoga, meditation and deep breathing.

DASH Diet (Dietary Approaches to Stop Hypertension): The DASH diet is rich in fruits, vegetables, whole grains, lean protein designed to lower blood pressure. You can control your blood pressure if you follow the DASH diet.

5.2 Exercise and Physical Activity

Exercising on a regular basis has many health benefits and protects people against high blood pressure and cardiovascular diseases. Studies show that by reducing systolic blood pressure by 5 mmHg, deaths from strokes can be reduced by 14% and deaths from coronary heart disease can be decreased by 9%. Regular exercise is key to preventing and treating hypertension. Physical inactivity among the adult population constitutes a real problem in the western region. Low levels of physical activity have a direct link with weight gain, which in turn increases the risk of raised blood pressure. In some countries of the region, the prevalence of physical inactivity can reach about 70% of the adult population. The situation among adolescents is not encouraging. Data on the combined risk factors of overweight and lack of physical activity show that adolescents do not exercise sufficiently.

There is a recommended amount of exercise by WHO for every age bracket for the prevention of chronic diseases such as cardiovascular diseases, stroke and hypertension.

Children and youth aged 5–17 years: Children should accumulate at least 60 minutes of moderate-to-vigorous intensity physical activity daily. Amounts of physical activity greater than 60 minutes provide additional health benefits.
Most of the daily physical activity should be aerobic. Vigorous intensity activities should be incorporated, including those that strengthen muscle and bone, at least 3 times per week.

Adults aged 18–64 years: Adults should accumulate at least 150 minutes of moderate intensity aerobic physical activity throughout the week or do at least 75 minutes of vigorous intensity aerobic physical activity throughout the week. For additional health benefits, adults should increase their moderate-intensity aerobic physical activity to 300 minutes per week, or engage in 150 minutes of vigorous intensity aerobic physical activity per week, or an equivalent combination of moderate and vigorous intensity activity. Muscle-strengthening activities should be carried out on 2 or more days a week.

Adults aged 65 years and older: Older adults should accumulate at least 150 minutes of moderate intensity aerobic physical activity throughout the week or do at least 75 minutes of vigorous intensity aerobic physical activity throughout the week. Aerobic activity should be performed in sessions of around 10-minutes duration. For additional health benefits, older adults should increase their moderate intensity aerobic physical activity to 300 minutes per week, or engage in 150 minutes of vigorous intensity aerobic physical activity per week.

Older adults with poor mobility should perform physical activity to enhance balance and prevent falls on 3 or more days per week.

Muscle-strengthening activities, involving major muscle groups, should be done on 2 or more days a week.

5.3 Stress Management and Hypertension

Do you notice how your body responds to stress? When you encounter a stressful situation, your body kicks into stress response mode. For example, if it's time to present the big slideshow you've been working on for months, your heart rate gets faster, and your blood pressure rises. And once the presentation is over, your body recovers, and blood pressure goes back to normal. But when you experience constant or chronic stress, your body is always on high alert. Your blood pressure may go up frequently. And over time, frequent blood pressure jumps can lead to hypertension (high blood pressure). Consistently elevated blood pressure can cause or worsen a range of health complications.

Fortunately, you can learn to cope with stress in healthy ways. First, know your stres triggers. Are there certain events, activities or situations that cause you stress? You can't always avoid your stress triggers, but you can prepare for them. Think about things that you can control and make a plan. You can lower your stress level by focusing on things within your power rather than things you can't control.

Second, put sleep on your schedule. When we're busy and stressed, sleep may get last place on the to-do list. But it should be one of the first things you focus on when you're overwhelmed. Inadequate or poor quality sleep can harm your mental alertness, mood, energy level and physical health. Getting quality sleep improves your mental and physical health, including your ability to deal with stress. Plus, when we sleep, our blood pressure drops. So a lack of quality sleep means your blood pressure stays higher for longer.

Third, be active. Moving your body helps you feel better mentally and can lower your blood pressure, too. Physical activity is a great way to manage hypertension and other heart conditions. You don't need expensive equipment or a gym membership to get active. Pick any activity that gets your heart rate up, such as walking, dancing or biking. Even a few minutes of exercise has stress relieving effects. Try to get 30 minutes of activity most days of the week. If you prefer, break it up into 10- or 15-minute chunks to fit your schedule.

Lastly, connect with people. Experts say nearly everyone can benefit from social support. Spending time with others in person or virtually can help you lower stress and improve your health. You can take a class to learn something new or volunteer with a nonprofit. And you don't need a huge circle of friends to feel connected. Having one trusted friend or family member to talk to can help you deal with life's challenges. Remember, you don't have to do this alone. Reach out to a neighbor or friend. If family stress feels overwhelming, hold a family meeting to discuss these issues. Together, you can discover ways everyone can lower their stress. Talk about ways to find balance between work and family demands.

Support groups are another way to connect with people who are dealing with similar challenges. Search online for support groups that fit your needs or ask your healthcare provider for recommendations.

5.4 Sleep and Blood Pressure

Sleep experts recommend that adults get 7 to 8 hours of sleep each night. Getting less than six hours of sleep is known to be bad for overall health. Stress, jet lag, shift work and other sleep disturbances make it more likely to develop heart disease and risk factors for heart disease, including obesity and diabetes. A regular lack of sleep may lead to high blood pressure (hypertension) in children and adults.

The less you sleep, the higher your blood pressure may go. People who sleep six hours or less may have steeper increases in blood pressure. If you already have high blood pressure, not sleeping well may make your blood pressure worse. It's thought that sleep helps the body control hormones needed to control stress and metabolism. Over time, a lack of sleep could cause swings in hormones. Hormone changes can lead to high blood pressure and other risk factors for heart disease. Don't try to make up for a lack of sleep with a lot of sleep. Too much sleep although not as bad as too little sleep can lead to high blood sugar and weight gain, which can affect heart health. Talk to your health care provider for tips on getting better sleep, especially if you have high blood pressure. One possible, treatable cause of lack of sleep contributing to high blood pressure is obstructive sleep apnea. This sleep disorder causes breathing to repeatedly stop and start during sleep. Talk with your care provider if you feel tired even after a full night's sleep, especially if you snore. Obstructive sleep apnea may be the cause. Obstructive sleep apnea can increase the risk of high blood pressure and other heart problems.

5.5 Reducing Alcohol and Sodium Intake

WHO has identified a set of evidence-based best buy interventions to tackle noncommunicable diseases that should be undertaken immediately, with expected accelerated results in terms of lives saved, healthy lives, life years gained, cases of disease prevented and costs avoided. There are 4 best buys for sodium reduction:

- the reformulation of food products to contain less salt and the setting of target levels for the amount of salt in foods and meals;
- the establishment of a supportive environment in public institutions such as hospitals, schools, workplaces and nursing homes to enable lower sodium options to be provided;
- the implementation of front-of-pack labeling; and
- behavior changes communication and mass media campaigns.

The development, implementation, monitoring and evaluation of sodium reduction policies should be government-led and safeguarded against possible conflicts of interest. WHO has developed a Sodium Country Score Card to monitor countries' progress in making national commitments and taking a multifaceted approach to implementing policies to reduce sodium intake.

That's WHO trying to reduce the salt intake, what about you. What can you do on your part to reduce your sodium intake?
- eat mostly fresh, minimally processed foods
- choose low-sodium products (less than 120 mg/100g sodium)
- cook with little or no added sodium/salt

- use herbs and spices to flavor food, rather than salt
- limit the use of commercial sauces, dressings and instant products
- limit the consumption of processed foods
- remove the salt shaker/container from the table.

Reducing alcohol intake is also necessary as a lifestyle modification. Now, alcohol is a common part of social gatherings, celebrations and daily life for many people. However, excessive consumption of alcohol can have adverse effects on both your mental and physical health thereby increasing your risk of high blood pressure. To reduce alcohol, you need to come out with strategies to help you make positive changes.

First, set realistic goals. A clear and achievable goal may be easier to maintain to reduce your intake.

Second, seek support. Talk to friends or family about your intention to reduce alcohol intake. Having a support system can help you stay on track.

Third, be mindful. This implies being conscious of your alcohol consumption. Keep track of the alcohol content and how many drinks you've had. This awareness can prevent overindulgence.

Furthermore, endeavor to find alternate coping strategies as many people turn to alcohol to help them cope with negative emotions or stress. Yours shouldn't be alcohol but exercise, meditation and things that make you happy.

Chapter 6: Medications and Treatment Options

6.1 Medications for Hypertension

The type of medicine used to treat hypertension depends on your overall health and how high your blood pressure is. Two or more blood pressure drugs often work better than one. It can take some time to find the medicine or combination of medicines that works best for you. When taking blood pressure medicine, it's important to know your goal blood pressure level. You should aim for a blood pressure treatment goal of less than 130/80 mm Hg if:

- You're a healthy adult age 65 or older
- You're a healthy adult younger than age 65 with a 10% or higher risk of developing cardiovascular disease in the next 10 years

- You have chronic kidney disease, diabetes or coronary artery disease.

The ideal blood pressure goal can vary with age and health conditions, particularly if you're older than age 65.

Medicines used to treat high blood pressure include:

Water Pills (diuretics): These drugs help remove sodium and water from the body. They are often the first medicines used to treat high blood pressure. There are different classes of diuretics, including thiazide, loop and potassium sparing. Which one your provider recommends depends on your blood pressure measurements and other health conditions, such as kidney disease or heart failure. Diuretics commonly used to treat blood pressure include chlorthalidone, hydrochlorothiazide (Microzide) and others. A common side effect of diuretics is increased urination. Urinating a lot can reduce potassium levels. A good balance of potassium is necessary to help the heart beat correctly. If you have low potassium (hypokalemia), your provider may recommend a potassium-sparing diuretic that contains triamterene.

Angiotensin-converting Enzyme (ACE) Inhibitors: These drugs help relax blood vessels. They block the formation of a natural chemical that narrows blood vessels. Examples include lisinopril (Prinivil, Zestril), benazepril (Lotensin), captopril and others.

Calcium channel blockers: These drugs help relax the muscles of the blood vessels. Some slow your heart rate. They include amlodipine

(Norvasc), diltiazem (Cardizem, Tiazac, others) and others. Calcium channel blockers may work better for older people and Black people than do angiotensin-converting enzyme (ACE) inhibitors alone. Don't eat or drink grapefruit products when taking calcium channel blockers. Grapefruit increases blood levels of certain calcium channel blockers, which can be dangerous. Talk to your provider or pharmacist if you're concerned about interactions.

There are other medicines sometimes used to treat high blood pressure. If you're having trouble reaching your blood pressure goal with combinations of the above medicines, your provider may prescribe:

Alpha Blockers: These medicines reduce nerve signals to blood vessels. They help lower the effects of natural chemicals that narrow blood vessels. Alpha blockers include doxazosin (Cardura), prazosin (Minipress) and others.

Alpha-beta Blockers: Alpha-beta blockers block nerve signals to blood vessels and slow the heartbeat. They reduce the amount of blood that must be pumped through the vessels. Alpha-beta blockers include carvedilol (Coreg) and labetalol (Trandate).

Beta Blockers: These medicines reduce the workload on the heart and widen the blood vessels. This helps the heart beat slower and with less force. Beta blockers include atenolol (Tenormin), metoprolol (Lopressor, Toprol-XL, Kapspargo sprinkle) and others. Beta blockers aren't usually recommended as the only medicine prescribed. They may work best when combined with other blood pressure drugs.

Aldosterone Antagonists: These drugs may be used to treat resistant hypertension. They block the effect of a natural chemical that can lead to salt and fluid buildup in the body. Examples are spironolactone (Aldactone) and eplerenone (Inspra).

Renin Inhibitors: Aliskiren (Tekturna) slows the production of renin, an enzyme produced by the kidneys that starts a chain of chemical steps that increases blood pressure. Due to a risk of serious complications, including stroke, you shouldn't take aliskiren with ACE inhibitors or ARBs.

Vasodilators: These medicines stop the muscles in the artery walls from tightening. This prevents the arteries from narrowing. Examples include hydralazine and minoxidil.

Central-acting Agents: These medicines prevent the brain from telling the nervous system to increase the heart rate and narrow the blood vessels. Examples include clonidine (Catapres, Kapvay), guanfacine (Intuniv) and methyldopa.

Always take blood pressure medicines as prescribed. Never skip a dose or abruptly stop taking blood pressure medicines. Suddenly stopping certain ones, such as beta blockers, can cause a sharp increase in blood pressure called rebound hypertension. If you skip doses because of cost, side effects or forgetfulness, talk to your care provider about solutions. Don't change your treatment without your provider's guidance.

6.2 Combination Therapies

Combination treatment means another class of blood pressure medication is added to the first drug to increase effectiveness. Many people with mild high blood pressure respond to one medication. It may take a few tries to find the most effective drug. However, sometimes one drug cannot control high blood pressure. The doctor may increase the dose or change the medication, yet the blood pressure stays high. That's when a second drug may be added.

Sometimes, patients with higher blood pressure need combination treatment -- even initially -- to bring it to a normal range. Combination treatment for hypertension is individualized. It gives the best possible control of blood pressure with the fewest side effects. Also, combination treatment may cost less. There may be less frequent doctor visits as the drug combination effectively manages the hypertension.

Thiazide diuretics may be used alone to treat hypertension. Low-dose diuretics, though, can also be used with other medications such as beta-blocker. When used in a drug combination, the diuretic has fewer side effects. It also boosts the blood-pressure-lowering effect of the other medication. Diuretics are added to other blood pressure medications. For instance, if the person with high blood pressure also retains fluid, a diuretic may be added.

ACE inhibitors or angiotensin receptor blockers are often effective when combined with other classes of medications. Sometimes, a beta-blocker is combined with an alpha-blocker. This may be useful for men who have hypertension and an enlarged prostate. The alpha-blocker may help both problems at the same time.

Other combinations may include an ACE inhibitor with a thiazide diuretic. Sometimes, an angiotensin II receptor antagonist is combined with a diuretic. Or an ACE inhibitor may be combined with a calcium channel blocker.

Your doctor will prescribe combination treatment cautiously. For instance, if both drugs lower the heart rate, your doctor will monitor you closely. This will keep you from having an excessively slow pulse (called bradycardia). If you have asthma, your doctor will avoid using drugs that could cause asthma-like symptoms. Trust your doctor to prescribe the most effective treatment with your health in mind.

6.3 Integrative and Alternative Approaches

While medication and lifestyle changes are the cornerstones of hypertension management, integrative and alternative approaches can complement traditional treatments. These strategies focus on holistic well-being and may contribute to blood pressure control. The following are some integrative and alternative approahes in hypertension treatment.

Mind-Body Practices: Chronic stress can elevate blood pressure. Mind-body practices such as mindfulness, meditation and yoga promote relaxation, reduces stress hormones and may help lower blood pressure. Incorporate these activities into your day to day life, even a few minutes of deep breathing and meditation can make a difference.

Acupuncture: This is an ancient Chinese practice which involves inserting thin needles into specific points on the body. Some studies say it may help lower blood pressure by balancing energy flow.

Biofeedback: This technique helps individuals control physiological functions such as blood pressure. It can also be used as a strategy to manage stress.

Dietary Supplements: Some dietary supplements help in the control of blood pressure such as potassium, magnesium and omega-3 fatty acids which have shown potential benefits. Despite their benefits, you're advice to contact you healthcare provider before taking them for determination of proper dosages.

Herbal Remedies: Some herbal remedies like garlic and hibiscus have this blood pressure lowering effect. Their efficacy varies and they can also interact with other medications.

Aromatherapy: Here, essential oils are use to boost relaxation and reduce stress. It may indirectly contribute to blood pressure control by mitigating stress.

Chiropractic: Spinal alignment and nerve function is improved through chiropractic adjustments. It may not be a direct treatment for hypertension but may have effects on overall wellbeing.

Exercise Therapies: Like we earlier discussed, exercise therapies like Tai chi and Qigong promotes physical and mental wellbeing thereby having a positive impact on stress reduction. These practices help in better blood pressure control.

Chapter 7: The DASH Diet: Dietary Approaches to Stop Hypertension

7.1 Understanding the DASH Diet

DASH stands for Dietary Approaches to Stop Hypertension. It is a healthy-eating plan designed to help prevent or treat high blood pressure, also called hypertension. It also may help lower cholesterol linked to heart disease, called low density lipoprotein (LDL) cholesterol.

The standard DASH diet limits salt to 2,300 milligrams (mg) a day. That amount agrees with the Dietary Guidelines for Americans. That's about the amount of sodium in 1 teaspoon of table salt. A lower sodium version of DASH restricts sodium to 1,500 mg a day. You can choose the version of the diet that meets your health needs. If you aren't sure what sodium level is right for you, talk to your health care provider.

7.2 Implementing the DASH Diet

The Dietary Approaches to Stop Hypertension is a well regarded dietary plan designed to help lower high blood pressure and generally improve cardiovascular health. Here's how one can implement the DASH diet for proper blood pressure control.

Emphasize Fruits and Vegetables: Fruits and vegetables are rich in nutrients which are very essential such as potassium and fiber which supports blood pressure control. Aim to consume lots of fruits and vegetables daily, fresh, frozen and canned (without added salt).

Choose Whole Grains: Whole grains such as brown rice, whole wheat and oat provides fiber and nutrients which are essential for blood pressure control. Opt for whole grain instead of refined grains in your bread, pasta, cereals and rice.

Include Lean Protein: Lean sources of protein have low saturated fat and can help lower blood pressure. They include fish, poultry and legumes. Choose skinless poultry, beans, lentils, peas and fatty fish like salmon and mackerel as your protein sources.

Moderate Diary Products: Low fat and fat free diary products are good source of calcium and potassium without the added saturated fat. Aim for low fat or fat free milk, yogurt and cheese in your diet. Lactose free options should be chosen if needed.

Reduce Sodium (Salt): Reducing excessive sodium intake can also help lower blood pressure as reducing salt is a fundamental aspect of the DASH diet.

Snack Smart: Healthy snacks provide essential nutrients and can also help curb hunger. Choose fruits, vegetables, unsalted nuts and whole grain snacks as a healthy snacking options.

Limit Sweets and Added Sugars: We all know what excess sugar can do, make you gain more weight and increase related health issues. Limit sugary foods and beverages in your diet, opt for natural sugars like honey or maple syrup as alternative.

Control Portion Sizes: Appropriate portion of food you take can help maintain a healthy weight which important for blood pressure control. Do not just consume food for the sake of it, use smaller plates to help cut down your food intake.

Plan Meals: Planning balanced meals in advance can help you adhere strictly to DASH diet and make healthy food choices.

Stay Hydrated: Being properly hydrated supports overall health and can help maintain healthy blood pressure levels.

Monitor Your Progress: Assessing your dietary choices regularly and tracking your progress can help you stay on the right path in controlling your blood pressure. Keep a good diary, measure sodium intake and measure your blood pressure regularly to gauge the effectiveness of the DASH diet.

7.3 Benefits and Potential Drawbacks

Following the DASH diet and staying physically active will provide the most significant benefit in lowering blood pressure. Here are the benefits:

Reduce High Blood Pressure: The origins of the DASH diet date back to the 90s when the NIH funded several studies to find a therapeutic diet effective at treating high blood pressure. They concluded that the DASH diet could lower blood pressure even without weight loss or intentional sodium restriction. Utilizing the DASH diet in conjunction with weight loss and sodium restriction can magnify blood pressure reductions.

Reduce High Cholesterol: The DASH diet is effective at improving markers of LDL and VLDL ("bad") cholesterol and triglycerides; however, the DASH diet also results in decreased HDL ("good") cholesterol. Further research has shown that a higher fat DASH diet, substituting 10% of total daily carbohydrates calories with unsaturated fat, is effective at lowering blood pressure, LDL cholesterol, and triglycerides to the same extent as the original DASH diet without resulting in unwanted reductions of HDL cholesterol.

Reduce Cardiovascular Diseases: Hypertension is a significant risk factor for most cardiovascular diseases, such as heart attack and stroke. Given its efficacy at lowering and normalizing blood pressure, the DASH diet can significantly protect against cardiovascular disease by 20%. Specifically, it is associated with a 19% lower risk of stroke and a 29% lower risk of heart failure.

Weight Loss: The DASH diet is a good choice for weight management, particularly for weight reduction in overweight and obese participants. A recent meta-analysis revealed that adults on the DASH diet lost more weight than those following a calorie-restricted standard American diet over 24 weeks.

Reduce Type 2 Diabetes: The DASH diet is associated with a 20% risk reduction in future type 2 diabetes. Insulin resistance, the desensitization of the body to insulin and the consequent rise in blood sugar, is a precursor to prediabetes and type 2 diabetes. The DASH diet effectively improves insulin sensitivity, especially when implemented as part of a comprehensive lifestyle modification program, including weight loss and exercise. Interestingly, utilizing glycemic index (GI) to make carbohydrate food choices on the DASH diet does not appear to be necessary, as both high- and low-GI DASH diets resulted in the same effects on insulin sensitivity.

Improve Metabolic Syndrome: Metabolic syndrome is the presence of at least three: high blood pressure, high blood sugar, abdominal obesity, low HDL cholesterol, and high triglycerides. Utilizing the DASH diet to improve these biomarkers can help prevent and manage metabolic syndrome.

Reduce Cancer Risk: Adherence to the DASH diet results in a lower risk of some cancers, including colorectal and breast cancer, due to its high content of vitamins, minerals, fiber, and antioxidants.

Reduce Gout Risk: Compared to a Standard American Diet, DASH can lower serum uric acid levels, translating to a lower risk of gout. With a popular understanding that gout is a metabolic disease, often co-occurring with high blood pressure and other cardiovascular diseases, the DASH diet would be helpful in addressing all conditions.

Improve Kidney Health: DASH dietary patterns of reduced consumption of red meat and processed foods and higher intake of nuts, legumes, and low-fat dairy products are associated with a lower risk of kidney disease. The affiliated high intake of calcium, phytates, magnesium, and citrate with eating fruits and vegetables on the DASH diet is also associated with decreased risk of kidney stones.

The DASH diet has its benefits and also its drawbacks. The following are the drawbacks:

*DASH requires each person to plan their own daily menus based on the allowed servings. People who are not used to meal planning or cooking may need more specific guidance.

* The types of foods listed are not comprehensive. For example, avocados are not included so it is not clear if they would be categorized as a fruit or a fat serving. Certain

foods are placed into questionable categories: pretzels are placed in the grain group even though they have fairly low nutrient content and no fiber; frozen yogurt is placed in the dairy group even though most brands contain little calcium and vitamin D and are high in added sugar. The general term "cereals" are placed in the grain group but different types of cereals can be highly variable in nutrient and sugar content.

- Those with lactose intolerance or food allergies (e.g., nuts) may need to modify the diet to include lactose-free alternatives to dairy and seeds instead of nuts.

- Some people may experience gas and bloating when starting the diet due to the high fiber content of plant foods like fruits, vegetables, and whole grains. This can be minimized by adding one or two new high fiber foods a week instead of all

at once.

Chapter 8: Monitoring and Selfcare

8.1 Keeping a Blood Pressure Journal

If you have high blood pressure, keeping a running log of blood pressure readings can help improve the quality of your treatment and highlight any special circumstances that may require additional intervention. Sometimes your healthcare provider will ask you to keep a blood pressure log to monitor how your pressures tend to vary during different times of the day or to see if your blood pressure shows any extreme spikes. Keeping a blood pressure log is not difficult and only takes three to five minutes per day. Measuring blood pressure will require a special device, and you may need to get training to learn how to use it properly. Your healthcare provider can help you with this training.

To keep a blood pressure log, you'll need to use a quality blood pressure monitor. The many different types and brands of blood pressure monitors on the market today vary in price. It's important to select one that provides a reliable and accurate reading. Blood pressure monitors may be digital or manual. A digital blood pressure monitor can be easier to use and offers less opportunity for error. Your healthcare provider can help you choose a reliable device.

Also, use standard measurement times. Because your blood pressure fluctuates during the day, keeping a blood pressure log will give the most accurate results if you always measure your blood pressure at the same time. Morning, afternoon and evening time are easy choices. The morning reading should be taken right after you wake up, and before you take any medicines, drink coffee or eat breakfast.

Keep a standardized record sheet that includes space for date, time, blood pressure reading, and notes. You should use the notes section to record information about any special circumstances that may be affecting your blood pressure during that reading. For example, if you took medicines before recording the reading. Any symptoms you may be experiencing at the time of the measurement should also be recorded in the notes section. You can download and print a standardized blood pressure log if you need one.

Take readings in a quiet place as recommended by the American Heart Association with both feet flat on the floor for 5 minutes before taking a blood pressure reading. Noise, distractions, and extremes in temperature can affect your blood pressure, as well as the accuracy of the reading. Taking the actual measurement is very simple once you've learned to use your blood pressure monitor, and it usually only takes 30 to 45 seconds. You simply attach a blood pressure cuff to your arm, press a button on the machine, and wait for the result to be displayed.

Record each reading immediately because they're easy to forget. If you get distracted and forget what the reading was, retake your blood pressure and write an explanatory note in the appropriate section of your log sheet.

Show the log sheet to your healthcare provider to explain any confusing readings on your log sheet and counsel you about what any trends in your blood pressure readings actually mean. They will also look to see your highest and lowest readings, when they occurred, and any symptoms you may have experienced at the time, such as headache, dizziness, or confusion.

8.2 Staying Compliant with Medications

In the treatment of hypertension, medications play a vital role in helping to lower and control blood pressure. The effectiveness of these medications rely heavily on consistency and pepper use. Staying compliant with your medication prescribed by the doctor helps for managing and controlling blood pressure. Below are tips to help you stay on track:

Understand your medications: First, you need to know what your medications do and why they were prescribed. Also, know the names of these medications, how they work and their side effects.

Follow the Prescribed Dosage: Taking the medication at the right time and dosage is crucial. Set reminders if needed.

Use Pill Organizers: This can help you keep track of your daily medication regimen.

Sync Medications with Daily Routines: Incorporate medications with your daily routine to make it a habit. Take your medication at the same time each day, aligning it with a routine task like brushing your teeth or having a meal.

Seek Combination Pills: Combining pills may break down your medication regimen by offering different medications in one dose. Discuss with your healthcare provider if combination pills are suitable for your needs and condition.

Communicate with Your Healthcare Provider: Communicating with your healthcare provider often can address any concerns or difficulties you have with your medication. If there are side effects or trouble affording your medication, do not hesitate to consult your healthcare provider.

Monitor Your Blood Pressure: These allow you to see the effectiveness of your medication and make adjustments where necessary. Keep the recordings of your blood pressure as recommended by your doctor.

Refill Prescriptions Promptly: Make sure you do not run out of medication as it may disrupt your treatment plan. Order refills in advance to avoid treatment gaps.

8.3 Regular Follow-ups and Adjustments

Once antihypertensive drug therapy is initiated, most patients should return for followup and adjustment of medications at monthly intervals or until the BP goal is reached. More frequent visits will be necessary for patients with stage 2 hypertension or with complicating comorbid conditions. Serum potassium and creatinine should be monitored at least one to two times per year. After BP is at goal and stable, followup visits can usually be at 3- to 6-month intervals. Comorbidities such as HF, associated diseases such as diabetes, and the need for laboratory tests influence the frequency of visits. Other cardiovascular risk factors should be monitored and treated to their respective goals, and tobacco avoidance must be promoted vigorously. Low-dose aspirin therapy should be considered only when BP is controlled because of the increased risk of hemorrhagic stroke when the hypertension is not controlled.

Chapter 9: Hypertension in Special Populations

9.1 High Blood Pressure in Children and Teens

High blood pressure in children varies based on their age, sex assigned at birth and height, as healthy blood pressure changes as your child grows. Children often don't have symptoms of high blood pressure, so it's important to take them to regular checkups with their healthcare provider. About 1 in 25 kids ages 12 to 19 have hypertension. About 1 in 10 has elevated blood pressure (formerly known as prehypertension).

High blood pressure is more common in boys and children assigned male at birth (AMAB) than girls and children assigned female at birth

(AFAB). It's also more common in Hispanic and non-Hispanic Black children compared to non-Hispanic white children. It is more common in children older than 12.

Over time, high blood pressure can damage a child's organs because their heart and blood vessels aren't delivering blood to their organs the way they should. This can damage a number of organs, including their heart, kidneys and eyes. Because of this, it's essential to diagnose and treat pediatric hypertension as soon as possible.

What are the symptoms of high blood pressure in children and teens?
While hypertension can cause symptoms in severe cases, most children with high blood pressure have no symptoms. Healthcare

providers usually discover it when checking a child's blood pressure during a routine checkup. This is one of the many reasons why it's important for your child to have regular medical checkups, especially if they have risk factors for high blood pressure.

What causes high blood pressure in children and teens?

There are two main types, or causes, of pediatric high blood pressure: primary hypertension and secondary hypertension.

Primary hypertension in children doesn't have one distinct cause. It's also known as idiopathic or essential hypertension. General characteristics of children with primary hypertension include: being age 6 or older, a family history of high blood pressure (biological parent or grandparent) and having overweight (a body mass index, or

BMI, greater than 25) or obesity (a BMI greater than 30). Primary hypertension is the most common form of high blood pressure in children.

For secondary hypertension in children, it happens when there is an underlying condition causing it. Kidney (renal) disease and renovascular disease (the narrowing of the artery to one or both kidneys) are the most common causes of secondary hypertension in children.

Other causes of pediatric secondary hypertension include: congenital heart conditions, such as aortic coarctation, hormonal imbalances (endocrine hypertension), like hyperthyroidism or catecholamine excess, obstructive sleep apnea, certain medications, common prescription medications associated with a rise in blood pressure include birth control pills, central nervous system stimulants and corticosteroids, genetic mutations (monogenic hypertension), such as Liddle syndrome or neurofibromatosis type 1, environmental exposures, including exposure to lead, cadmium, mercury and phthalates.

9.2 Hypertension in Pregnancy

High blood pressure in pregnancy has become more common. However, with good blood pressure control, you and your baby are more likely to stay healthy. The most important thing to do is talk with your health care team about any blood pressure problems so you can get the right treatment and control your blood pressure before you get pregnant. Getting treatment for high blood pressure is important before, during, and after pregnancy.

There are complications from high pressure during pregnancy. For the mother, preeclampsia, eclampsia, stroke, the need for labor induction (giving medicine to start labor to give birth), and placental abruption (the placenta separating from the wall of the uterus) while for the baby, the complications are preterm delivery (birth that happens before 37 weeks of pregnancy) and low birth weight (when a baby is born weighing less than 5 pounds, 8 ounces). The mother's high blood pressure makes it more difficult for the baby to get enough oxygen and nutrients to grow, so the mother may have to deliver the baby early.

What should you do if you have high blood pressure before, during or after pregnancy?

Before pregnancy, make a plan for pregnancy and talk with your doctor or health care team about the following:

- Any health problems you have or had and any medicines you are taking. If you are planning to become pregnant, talk to your doctor. Your doctor or health care team can help you find medicines that are safe to take during pregnancy.
- Ways to keep a healthy weight through healthy eating and regular physical activity.

During Pregnancy:

- Get early and regular prenatal care. Go to every appointment with your doctor or health care professional.

- Talk to your doctor about any medicines you take and which ones are safe. Do not stop or start taking any type of medicine, including over-the-counter medicines, without first talking with your doctor.

- Keep track of your blood pressure at home with a home blood pressure monitor. Contact your doctor if your blood pressure is higher than usual or if you have symptoms of preeclampsia. Talk to your doctor or insurance company about getting a home monitor.

- Continue to choose healthy foods and keep a healthy weight.

After Pregnancy:

- Pay attention to how you feel after you give birth. If you had high blood pressure during pregnancy, you have a higher risk for stroke and other problems after delivery. Tell your doctor or call 9-1-1 right away if you have symptoms of preeclampsia after delivery. You might need emergency medical care.

9.3 Managing Hypertension in Older Adults

Encouraging healthy aging and reducing the risk of cardiovascular diseases need proper management of hypertension, also referred to as high blood pressure. A prevalent problem among the elderly is hypertension. Because the cardiovascular health of older adults can be significantly impacted by age-related changes, regular blood pressure monitoring is crucial. Personalized blood pressure goals should be considered while treating hypertension in the elderly, since these can vary based on the general health and medical history of the patient.

Medication schedules may need to be adjusted over time to take potential drug interactions and aging-related changes into consideration. Elderly people frequently have a polypharmacy habit, which can make it more difficult to control their hypertension.

Additionally, because they may be more vulnerable to drug side effects, older folks should be on the lookout for any possible ones. Because medication adherence can be impacted by memory and cognitive function, it is crucial to monitor cognitive health. Older persons can employ pill organizers, reminders, or caregiver assistance to support adherence.

Support and guidance in controlling hypertension can be obtained from a robust network of social connections. People can stay compliant with their medicine and lead heart-healthy lives by involving friends, family, or support groups.

Controlling blood pressure and heart health also depend on physical activity. Respecting their physical limitations, older adults should engage in regular, low-impact exercise. Nutrition is important, and managing hypertension can be aided by eating a balanced diet rich in fruits, vegetables, whole grains, lean meats, and low-fat dairy products. It is particularly crucial to reduce added sugars and salt.

Regular check-ups with medical professionals enable the early identification and treatment of hypertension and other health problems. Frequent visits assist in addressing any issues or symptoms, reviewing medications, and monitoring blood pressure.

Lastly, two crucial aspects of managing hypertension are stress management and preserving mental health. A person's general well-being is enhanced by relaxing regularly, having fun, and getting emotional support when required.

Finally, it should be noted that older adults have to efficiently handle their hypertension in order to promote healthy aging and reduce the likelihood of cardiovascular problems. Through individualized care, medication management, lifestyle modifications, routine checkups, and support networks, it ultimately enables older adults to lead happy, healthy lives as they age.

Chapter 10: Blood Pressure and Your Health

10.1 Heart-Healthy Habits

Adopting healthy habits can be your best defense against heart disease, and may also help prevent heart attack and stroke. Here are some of the best things you can do for a healthier heart:

Make Exercise a Regular Part of Your Life: Your heart is a muscle, and just like pecs or abs, it needs to be worked out consistently to stay strong. Doing aerobic exercise most days of the week for 30 to 60 minutes will help keep your heart working as efficiently as possible. If you're looking to lose some weight, add some light weight training for an additional metabolic kick.

Keep Your Diet in Balance: Meals aren't just fuel. Food can be medicine. Eating right for your heart means building meals on a foundation of whole grains, fruits and veggies, adding low-fat dairy, poultry, fish and nuts to round out your diet. Limit or avoid red meat, processed foods and foods high in sodium. Remember to drink plenty of fluids every day and consider adding green tea if you enjoy the taste. Certain foods and some dietary supplements may help to decrease inflammation and cholesterol and improve high blood pressure. These include artichoke, garlic, fish oil, magnesium, coenzyme Q10 and fiber.

Keep Your Blood Pressure in Check: High blood pressure, also known as hypertension, is a major risk factor when it comes to heart disease. If you can keep your blood pressure within a healthy range, that will reduce strain on your heart and arteries. Regular exercise and a healthy diet will help keep your blood pressure in check. Limiting alcohol and avoiding tobacco smoke are also important when it comes to managing blood pressure, as well as managing stress. Try incorporating meditation techniques through activities, such as yoga and tai chi for stress management.

Work on Loosing Weight if You Need to: Carrying around too much weight puts you at a higher risk for many health problems, including heart disease. Come up with a smart and realistic weight loss plan, approach it systematically and stick to your plan. Most importantly, when you've reached your goal, create a vigilant maintenance plan so you won't have to go through the process all over again.

Get Enough Regular Sleep Each Night: Good quality sleep is essential to health and well-being. Your heart is significantly impacted when your body doesn't get enough sleep. Just as your body needs rest, so does your heart. Most people need six to eight hours of sleep each day. If you're having problems falling or staying asleep, talk to your doctor to rule out a sleep disorder. There are many things you can do on your own to sleep better and feel better.

10.2 Blood Pressure and Heart Disease Prevention

Heart disease, still one of the most prevalent and deadly medical conditions, is largely predisposed by high blood pressure, or hypertension. For effective prevention, it is essential to comprehend the link between high blood pressure and heart disease. An extensive guide on how controlling blood pressure can help avoid heart disease is provided here:

Blood Pressure Management as a Proactive Approach: An important part of preventing heart disease is controlling blood pressure. It lessens the chance of harm to the arteries, heart, and other organs.

Changes in Lifestyle: Making lifestyle adjustments can be a very effective way to lower blood pressure and prevent heart disease. A heart-healthy diet, frequent exercise, giving up smoking, and moderation in alcohol intake are a few of these.

Dietary Selections: A diet low in saturated and trans fats, cholesterol, and sodium is characterized by an emphasis on fruits, vegetables, whole grains, lean proteins, and low-fat dairy products. In addition to lowering the risk of heart disease, this diet can help control blood pressure.

Workout Routine: To maintain a healthy weight, lower stress levels, and enhance general cardiovascular health, regular physical activity is essential. Aim for 150 minutes or more a week of moderate-to-intense exercise.

Giving Up Smoking: Smoking raises blood pressure, damages blood vessels, and dramatically increases the risk of heart disease. One of the biggest preventative measures against heart disease is to stop smoking.

Moderation with Alcohol: Heart disease and elevated blood pressure can result from excessive alcohol consumption. If you choose to drink, do so in moderation.

Management of Medication: To regulate blood pressure, some people may need to take medication. Effective management of hypertension requires consistent adherence to prescribed medication regimen and close collaboration with a healthcare provider.

Consistently checking blood pressure: For the early detection and management of hypertension, routine blood pressure checks are essential. Monitoring blood pressure at home with a blood pressure monitor can also be helpful in the long run.

Handling Stress: Long-term stress raises blood pressure and is linked to heart disease. Stress-reduction methods including deep breathing, meditation, and relaxation exercises can be effective strategies for lowering blood pressure and preventing heart disease.

Controlling Weight: Blood pressure is lowered and the risk of heart disease is decreased when one maintains a healthy weight. A diet and exercise regimen combined is essential for achieving and sustaining a good weight.

Sleep Guidance: Elevated blood pressure and an elevated risk of heart disease can result from inadequate sleep. Making proper sleep hygiene a priority is essential for maintaining cardiovascular health in general and controlling blood pressure.

Consistent Health Examinations: A healthcare provider's comprehensive health examinations can monitor your blood pressure and other vital signs and help determine your risk of heart disease.

Compliance with Medication: Following a doctor's prescription closely is crucial for achieving successful blood pressure management if medication is recommended to treat hypertension.

Chapter 11: Beyond Hypertension

11.1 Hypertension and Other Health Conditions

When your blood pressure is high for too long, it damages your blood vessels – and LDL (bad) cholesterol begins to accumulate along tears in your artery walls. This leads to narrowed arteries and increases the workload of your circulatory system while decreasing its efficiency. As a result, high blood pressure puts you at greater risk for developing life-changing and life-threating conditions. In most cases, damage done from high blood pressure (HBP or hypertension) occurs over time. Left undetected or uncontrolled, high blood pressure can lead to:

Heart Attack: High blood pressure damages arteries that can become blocked and prevent blood flow to the heart muscle.

Stroke: High blood pressure can cause blood vessels that supply blood and oxygen to the brain to become blocked or burst.

Heart Failure: The increased workload from high blood pressure can cause the heart to enlarge and fail to supply blood to the body.

Kidney Disease or Failure: High blood pressure can damage the arteries around the kidneys and interfere with their ability to filter blood effectively.

Vision Loss: High blood pressure can strain or damage blood vessels in the eyes.

Sexual Dysfunction: High blood pressure can lead to erectile dysfunction in men and may contribute to lower libido in women.

Angina: Over time, high blood pressure can lead to heart disease including microvascular disease (MVD). Angina, or chest pain, is a common symptom.

Peripheral Artery Disease (PAD): Atherosclerosis caused by high blood pressure can lead to narrowed arteries in the legs, arms, stomach and head, causing pain or fatigue.

11.2 Taking Charge of Your Overall Health

We rely on doctors and other providers to diagnose and treat medical conditions, but the most important person in your health care is you.

We can't completely control our health, but there are things that we can take charge of that will make a positive difference. By starting with a few small changes, you'll gain a sense of control quickly.

Keep Track of Your Health Information: Keep a written record of your health, a current list of prescriptions and supplements that you take; when your doctor wants you to report any measurements you make at home such as your weight, blood pressure, or blood sugar; when each of your last screening tests was done. Doctors who use electronic health records can print these out for you. Your individual targets for measurements made at home may vary depending on your age and overall health, but for most adults blood pressure should be less than 120/80 mm Hg. You're considered to have impaired fasting glucose, part of the definition of prediabetes, if your fasting glucose level is between 100 and 125 mg/dL. And your cholesterol levels are in the healthy range if the HDL is above 40 mg/dL and the LDL is below 100 mg/dL.

Don't Miss Your Screening Tests: Your doctor should set targets for how often you need different screening tests. Check with your doctor if you think you're due for a test. See our chart on this page for general recommendations.

Speak Up About Your Health: Ask questions and state preferences when it comes to treatment. Share new symptoms in detail with your physician. And if your doctor orders tests, here are some important questions to ask: What do you think the symptoms indicate? Why is this test necessary? What therapies are available? What is the prognosis? Are there any additional costs beyond my anticipated insurance reimbursement?

Get Moving: Regular exercise has more power to protect your health than any medicine ever invented. It reduces your resting heart rate, and allows your heart to work more efficiently. Exercise also lowers blood pressure and improves your cholesterol and the way you process blood. That can help prevent heart disease, stroke, and some forms of dementia. Exercise also causes nerve cells to release proteins called neurotrophic factors. Research in lab animals has shown these proteins stimulate the growth of new brain cells, improve neural connections in the brain, and help to regulate metabolism, energy, and mood. Exercise may also delay cognitive decline. Strive for at least 150 minutes per week of moderate-intensity exercise, such as brisk walking. If you're unable to get aerobic exercise because of a health condition, weight lifting has also been shown to be effective at staving off diabetes and osteoporosis.

Eat Your Way to Good Health: Get rid of the junk—saturated fats, high-sodium foods, and prepackaged foods. Replace them with fresh, natural food. Take at least 4½ cups of vegetables and fruits a day, including dark leafy greens, and anything that's a rich yellow, orange, or red color, such as tomatoes, oranges, strawberries, red peppers, sweet potatoes, carrots, and bananas. The Centers for Disease Control recommends keeping protein to 10% to 35% of your daily diet, and of that, the healthiest sources of proteins include lean meats, poultry, and fish, and plant-based proteins, such as nuts and beans.

Your diet is also linked to your weight, and maintaining a healthy weight has a direct impact on your health. Weight loss is good for your blood pressure and your cholesterol, for processing glucose and insulin, and for reducing inflammation and relieving joint pain.

Chapter 12: The Road to Hypertension Control

12.1 Setting Realistic Goals

On the journey to hypertension control, setting realistic goals is one step in enhancing your chances of success. Here's a guide on how you can achieve objectives that align with your pursuit of blood pressure control:

Understand Your Current Status: In setting realistic goals, first, you need to have a clear understanding of your current blood pressure levels and overall health. Monitoring your blood pressure regularly and a comprehensive health assessment will provide the necessary insights.

Define Specific Blood Pressure Targets: Your specific blood pressure objectives should be clear. For example, instead of a vague goal like "lowering blood pressure, " set a more realistic target like reduce systolic blood pressure from 150 to 130 mm Hg."

Apply the S.M.A.R.T. Framework: Utilize the S.M.A.R.T. criteria to structure your goals:

- Specific: clearly write down what you want to achieve regarding your blood pressure.

- Measurable: Define how your progress and success will be measured.

- Achievable: Based on your medical history and circumstances, ensure your goals are attainable and realistic.

- Relevant: Your goals should have a relationship with hypertension control and your overall health.
- Time-bound: In achieving your blood pressure target, set a timeline, creating a sense of urgency.

Start Gradually: Begin with smaller and manageable changes in your lifestyle and meditation routine. For example, learn to reduce sodium intake by a certain amount or take a daily work.

Focus on Lifestyle Adjustments: Prioritize changes in your diet, exercise, stress management and sleep patterns as many hypertension goals revolve around lifestyle.

Seek Professional Guidance: Consult a healthcare provider as they can offer insights, advice and guidance in setting realistic blood pressure goals.

Break Goals into Milestones: Your overarching blood pressure goals should be divided into smaller milestones. For example, if your ultimate target is to lower your blood pressure by 20 points, set milestones to track your progress, such as aiming for a 5-point reduction every few months.

Be Consistent: You can only achieve these goals if you're consistent as consistency is key. Develop daily or weekly routines that support your goals and maintain them.

Stay Flexible: Be ready to adapt and open to adjustments in whatever life may throw at you without loosing sight of your objectives.

Monitor Progress: Record your blood pressure readings, lifestyle changes and medication adherence as data will help track your progress and make informed decisions.

Celebrate Achievements: Recognize and celebrate what you have achieved so far no matter how small they may seem.

Learn from Setbacks: Setbacks may occur but view them as an opportunity to learn and improve. Analyze the reasons behind the setback and use that information to make adjustments.

Stay Motivated: Keep your motivation high by reminding yourself of the benefits of achieving your goals. Visualize a healthier, happier life as a result of your efforts.

Share Your Goals: Sharing your blood pressure control goals with trusted individuals, such as friends or family, can provide a support system that encourages accountability and offers motivation.

12.2 Overcoming Challenges

The journey through hypertension control may have challenges but with determination and the necessary strategies you can overcome these barriers and achieve your blood pressure management goal.

First, you have to be adherent to medications. Being consistent with prescribed medications might be difficult especially with its cost and effects on you. Try not to be forgetful too.

Adopting and maintaining a healthier lifestyle may also be challenging especially when you're faced with old routines. Remember, you do not have to change your lifestyle at once, a gradual change may be helpful so it doesn't get tiring. You can tell a friend or family member to help you out so you can make these changes gradually especially when it comes to diet and exercising your body.

For stress management, we've talked about how not managing your stress can increase your blood pressure. We said earlier you need relaxation techniques such as yoga, mindfulness and deep breathing. Believe me, when you take all these lightly it may no longer be challenging.

Monitoring your blood pressure and weight may be cumbersome and may require long term commitment respectively. Patience is key, you'll win this battle. Ensure to talk to your healthcare provider concerning the challenges you may be facing for advice.

12.3 Celebrating Successes

Celebrating successes is very important and often overlooked after your achievements whether big or small in hypertension control. These celebrations can boost your motivation and reinforce your commitment in managing your blood pressure effectively. There are so many reasons you have to celebrate your achievements. Through your successes you get motivated to continue working towards your hypertension control goals, positive reinforcement to make you maintain healthy behaviors, reduction in stress and anxiety which benefits your overall health and a sense of achievement which boost self esteem and confidence.

How do you celebrate these successes? Celebrations can come in any form and the key is to choose what is enjoyable and meaningful to you. You could go out with your friends to spend time together. Remember, you still need to be conscious not to engage in things that could ruin your successes.